Emergency Triage

Rapid Assessment and Prioritization in Critical Care Settings

Robin R. Vandyne, RN, MSN, CEN

Copyright © 2024 by Robin R. Vandyne, RN, MSN, CEN

All rights reserved. No part of this book may be reproduced, stored in a retrieval system, or transmitted in any form or by any means, including electronic, mechanical, photocopying, recording, or otherwise, without the prior written permission of the publisher, except for brief quotations used in reviews or academic works as permitted by copyright law.

Acknowledgements

I extend my heartfelt gratitude to everyone who contributed to the creation of this book. To my colleagues and mentors, whose insights and expertise provided invaluable guidance throughout this journey, thank you for inspiring me to explore and refine these concepts. To my family and friends, your unwavering support and encouragement have been my anchor, enabling me to pursue this work with dedication and focus.

I also acknowledge the countless healthcare professionals whose tireless efforts in the field continue to drive innovation and excellence in patient care. Your commitment to improving lives served as a profound source of inspiration for this project.

Finally, I am grateful to my readers, whose curiosity and passion for knowledge motivated me to create a resource that is both practical and impactful. This book is a testament to our shared pursuit of excellence in healthcare.

Preface

Emergency medicine is a field where every second counts. The ability to assess, prioritize, and respond to critical situations with precision and confidence is the cornerstone of effective patient care. Emergency Triage: Rapid Assessment and Prioritization in Critical Care Settings was written to provide healthcare professionals with a practical and streamlined guide to navigating the complexities of triage in diverse emergency settings.

This book is designed for nurses, paramedics, physicians, and other emergency care providers who are on the front lines of saving lives. It delivers clear, evidence-based approaches to evaluating patients, making rapid decisions, and allocating resources effectively in high-pressure environments. Grounded in real-world experience and clinical expertise, the content bridges the gap between theoretical knowledge and practical application.

Key features of this book include:

Comprehensive Triage Frameworks: Structured protocols for initial patient assessment and prioritization, covering diverse emergencies such as trauma, cardiac events, respiratory distress, and mass casualty scenarios.

Critical Thinking Tools: Strategies to sharpen decision-making skills and prioritize care when faced with competing demands.

Real-World Case Studies: Illustrative examples and case scenarios to help readers contextualize principles and apply them in practice.

Simplified Explanations: Clear and concise discussions of critical concepts, making the material accessible to learners at all levels.

Multidisciplinary Insights: Contributions from nursing, medical, and allied health perspectives, emphasizing collaborative teamwork in emergency care.

As an emergency nurse and educator at Manchester Royal Infirmary, I have witnessed firsthand the challenges and triumphs of triage. This book is a culmination of years of clinical practice, education, and research, aimed at equipping healthcare providers with the tools they need to deliver optimal care under pressure.

Whether you are a seasoned practitioner or new to the field, Emergency Triage: Rapid Assessment and Prioritization in Critical Care Settings will serve as a valuable resource. My hope is that this book not only enhances your clinical skills but also inspires confidence in your ability to make a difference during life's most critical moments.

Thank you for choosing this book as part of your professional journey. Together, we can ensure that every patient receives the timely and effective care they deserve.

Sincerely,
Robin R. Vandyne, RN, MSN, CEN
Emergency Nurse Educator
Manchester Royal Infirmary

Acknowledgement
Preface
Table of Content

Table of contents

Chapter 1: Introduction to Emergency Triage

1. Overview of Triage Systems
    - Importance of Triage in Emergency Care
    - Addressing Resource Constraints and Clinical Demand

2. Historical Evolution of Triage Practices
    - Early Intuitive Methods
    - Need for Standardization

3. Formation of the Manchester Triage Group
    - Objectives of the Group

- Development of a Standardized Framework

4. The Five-Level Triage System
    - Categories, Colors, and Maximum Response Times
    - Universal Adaptability of the System

5. Triage Methodology
    - Assigning Clinical Priority
    - The Flowchart-Guided Process

6. Differentiating Clinical Priority and Clinical Management
    - Balancing Urgency with Resource Allocation
    - Factors Influencing Management Decisions

7. Training and Auditing for Triage Implementation
    - Structured Training Programs
    - Sentinel Diagnoses and Retrospective Reviews

8. Applications Beyond Emergency Departments
    - Triage in Primary Care and Telephone Consultations
    - Integration with Dynamic Monitoring Tools

9. Summary of Triage Principles
    - Standardized Methodology for Effective Emergency Care
    - The Role of Triage in Improving Patient Outcomes

Chapter 2: The Decision-Making Process and Triage

1. Introduction to Decision-Making in Clinical Practice
    - Importance of Structured Decision-Making
    - Challenges of Unstructured Approaches

2. Historical Evolution of Triage Decision-Making
    - The SOAPE Assessment Tool
    - Transition to Standardized Frameworks

3. Developing Clinical Expertise
    - Five Stages of Expertise Development:
    - Novice
    - Advanced Beginner
    - Competent
    - Proficient
    - Expert

4. Key Decision-Making Strategies
    - Inductive and Deductive Reasoning
    - Pattern Recognition in Clinical Contexts
    - Repetitive Hypothesizing
    - Mental Representation of Complex Scenarios
    - Role of Intuition in Clinical Practice

5. Structured Decision-Making in Triage
    - The Five Phases of Triage Decision-Making:
    - Problem Identification
    - Information Gathering and Analysis
    - Evaluation and Selection of Alternatives
    - Implementation of Decisions
    - Monitoring and Reassessment

6. Overcoming Challenges in Adopting Standardized Frameworks
    - Resistance from Experienced Practitioners
    - Benefits of Standardization for Teaching and Auditing

7. Adapting the Framework to Diverse Practice Settings
    - Application Across Various Clinical Environments
    - Enhancing Reliability and Quality in Patient Care

Chapter 3: The Triage Method

1. Introduction
   - Overview of the Triage Method
   - Prioritization Based on Symptoms

2. Identifying the Problem
   - Importance of Presenting Complaints
   - Comprehensive List of Common Presentations

3. Gathering and Analyzing Information
   - Selecting Flowcharts for Presenting Complaints
   - Key Discriminators in Triage
   - General Discriminators
   - Specific Discriminators

4. General Discriminators
   - Life Threat
   - Hemorrhage
   - Pain
   - Conscious Level
   - Temperature

- Acuteness

5. Secondary Triage
    - Role in High-Volume Settings
    - Refining Clinical Priorities

6. Triage Activity Assessment
    - Initial Observation
    - Greeting the Patient
    - Assessing Visual Signs and Mobility
    - Patient History
    - Determining the Presenting Complaint
    - Focused Questions for In-Depth Assessment
    - Physical Examination and Parameters

7. Pain Assessment
    - Subjective and Objective Pain Scoring
    - Addressing Discrepancies

8. Priority and Plan of Care
    - Assigning Clinical Priority
    - Immediate Care Recommendations

9. Documentation
    - Key Information to Record
    - Maintaining Patient Focus During Digital Entry

10. Reassessment and Monitoring
    - Importance of Dynamic Re-Evaluation
    - Tracking Changes in Clinical Priority

11. Conclusion
    - Benefits of Structured Triage Methodology
    - Continuous Monitoring for Quality Care

Chapter 4: Pain Assessment as Part of the Triage Process

1. Introduction
    - Importance of Pain Assessment in the Emergency Department (ED)
    - Challenges of Oligoanalgesia
    - Benefits of Incorporating Pain Assessment into Triage

2. Pain Assessment Process in Triage
    - Role of Pain in the Manchester Triage System
    - Principles of Effective Pain Assessment

3. Challenges of Pain Assessment in Emergency Settings
    - Subjectivity of Pain Reporting
    - Traditional Practices and Biases
    - Misuse of Pain Scales

4. Pain Assessment Tools
    - Verbal Descriptor Scales
    - Visual Analogue Scales (VAS)
    - Pain Behavior Tools

5. The Ideal Pain Assessment Tool
    - Criteria for Effectiveness in EDs
    - Overview of the Pain Ruler
    - Supplementary Tools for Specific Populations

6. Key Considerations in Triage Pain Assessment
    - Age-Specific Pain Perceptions (Children and Elderly)
    - Influence of Previous Pain Experiences
    - Cultural and Social Norms
    - Role of Anxiety in Pain Perception
    - Impact of Pain on Daily Activities
    - Special Populations and Alternative Assessment Methods

7. Conclusion
    - Importance of Skilled Pain Assessment in the ED
    - Addressing Challenges for Improved Patient Outcomes

Chapter 5: Patient Management, Triage, and the Role of the Triage Nurse

1. Introduction
    - Importance of Effective Triage in the Emergency Department (ED)

- Clinical and Non-Clinical Factors Influencing Patient Management

2. Patient-Specific Considerations
   - Children: Managing Distress and Providing Comfort
   - Elderly Patients: Addressing Mobility, Anxiety, and Special Needs
   - Patients with Disabilities or Learning Difficulties: Ensuring Equitable Care
   - Aggressive or Abusive Patients: Strategies for Safety and Efficiency
   - Patients Under the Influence of Alcohol: Challenges and Reassessment
   - Frequent Visitors (Regulars): Recognizing Underlying Health Risks
   - Re-Attending Patients: Prioritizing Current Symptoms
   - Clinic Patients and Referrals: Streamlining Care Coordination

3. Departmental Dynamics

- Overcrowding and Resource Management: Strategies for Optimal Workflow
- Fast-Tracking and Streaming: Aligning Care Pathways with Patient Needs
- Managing Quiet Periods: Maintaining Momentum and Preventing Delays

4. Role of the Triage Nurse
    - Key Responsibilities: Prioritization and Decision-Making
    - First Aid and Pain Management: Immediate Interventions
    - Health Promotion: Enhancing Preventive Care
    - Dynamic Patient Reassessment: Ongoing Triage Responsibilities

5. Optimizing ED Flow
    - Patient Placement: Enhancing Comfort and Efficiency
    - Waiting Room Management: Observation, Communication, and Safety

6. Conclusion
    - Comprehensive, Patient-Centered Approaches to Triage
    - Balancing Clinical and Operational Priorities for High-Quality Care

Chapter 6: Auditing the Triage Process

1. Introduction
    - Importance of Auditing in the Manchester Triage System (MTS)
    - Ensuring Consistency and Quality in Triage Decisions

2. Audit Methodology
    - Identifying Practitioners and Triage Episodes
    - Random Sampling and Episode Assessment
    - Evaluation Metrics: Completeness and Accuracy
    - Feedback Mechanisms and Continuous Quality Improvement

- Frequency and Scalability of Audits

3. Key Criteria for Assessment
    - Use of Presentation Flowcharts
    - Accurate Documentation of Discriminators and Pain Scores
    - Assignment of Triage Categories and Record Legibility
    - Re-Triage Procedures

4. Defining Completeness and Accuracy
    - Completeness: Essential Steps and Common Omissions
    - Accuracy: Alignment of Presentation, Discriminator, and Condition

5. Practical Impact of Audits
    - Improvements in Documentation and Compliance
    - Addressing Common Errors and Enhancing Practitioner Performance

6. Case Studies and Global Findings

- Regional Audit in England: Variations in Accuracy and Case Mix
- National Audit in Portugal: Implementation and Outcomes

7. Conclusion
   - Role of Audits in Quality Assurance and Risk Management
   - Driving Improvements in Triage Practices Globally

Chapter 7: Telephone Triage

1. Introduction
   - Origins and Evolution of Telephone Triage
   - Benefits in Emergency Care Settings
   - Telephone Advice vs. Telephone Triage

2. Telephone Triage Methodology
   - Clinical Priority and Symptom-Based Assessment

- Outcome Categories: Medicine Now, Medicine Soon, Medicine Later
- Role of Local Service Information

3. Decision-Making Process
    - Information Gathering and Flowchart Selection
    - Evaluating Discriminators for Symptom Assessment
    - Tailoring Questions to Telephone-Based Triage

4. Interim Advice
    - Providing Stabilization Measures
    - Examples for Common Emergency Scenarios

5. Pain Assessment in Telephone Triage
    - Challenges in Remote Pain Evaluation
    - Using Pain as a Discriminator in Prioritization

6. Role of the Telephone Triage Practitioner
    - Essential Skills and Clinical Judgment

- Importance of Protocols, Flowcharts, and Continuous Training

7. Conclusion
   - Structured and Auditable Patient Prioritization
   - Ensuring Safety and Efficiency in Remote Emergency Care

Chapter 8: Beyond Prioritization

1. Introduction
   - Evolution of the Triage System
   - Extending Applications Beyond Prioritization

2. Dynamic Monitoring
   - Importance of Periodic Reassessments
   - Early Warning Score Systems vs. Triage Discriminators
   - Key Discriminators and Actions
   - Red, Orange, and Yellow Indicators

3. Presentation-Priority Matrix Mapping
    - Concept and Purpose of the Matrix
    - Matrix Utilization for Patient Disposition
    - Defined Dispositions
    - Handling Grey Areas
    - Adapting to Local Variability
    - Future Implications for Emergency Care

4. Extended Functions of Triage Consultations
    - Pain Management
    - Direct Referrals for Imaging and Specialist Care
    - Pathway Initiation for Self-Care and Primary Care
    - Benefits of Extended Triage Functions
    - Improved Patient Experience
    - Streamlined Processes
    - Efficient Resource Use
    - Challenges and Solutions
    - Managing Increased Consultation Times

- Addressing Training Needs

5. Conclusion
    - Advancing the Role of Triage in Modern Healthcare
    - Evidence-Based Implementation and Resource Optimization

Differentiation Glossary

Chapter 1
Introduction to Emergency Triage

Triage is a critical system of clinical risk management utilized across emergency departments worldwide to ensure efficient and safe patient care when clinical demand surpasses available resources. Its primary goal is to prioritize care based on clinical urgency, ensuring patients receive treatment according to their immediate needs. Historically, triage was an intuitive and inconsistent practice, lacking a standardized, auditable, and reproducible methodology.

To address these gaps, the Manchester Triage Group was established in November 1994. This multidisciplinary group of emergency physicians and nurses aimed to standardize triage practices, resulting in five key objectives:

1. Development of unified terminology.

2. Creation of consistent definitions.

3. Design of a reliable triage methodology.

4. Implementation of a structured training program.

5. Establishment of an audit framework to evaluate triage effectiveness.

Evolution of Triage Nomenclature and Definitions

A review of existing triage systems revealed significant variation in nomenclature and definitions. Common themes, however, emerged across different systems, enabling the development of a new standardized model. This model introduced five triage categories, each defined by a number, color, and a maximum ideal time to first clinical contact:

Category	Colour	Maximum Time (Minutes)
Immediate	Red	0
Very urgent	Orange	10
Urgent	Yellow	60
Standard	Green	120
Non - urgent	Blue	220

This five-level triage scale, now widely adopted, allows local adaptation while maintaining a universal framework to address clinical priority.

Triage Methodology

The Manchester Triage Method focuses on assigning clinical priority rather than providing a diagnosis or disposition. This approach ensures that emergency department operations and individual patient management are optimized. The methodology requires practitioners to:

1. Identify the patient's presentation.

2. Evaluate specific signs and symptoms (termed discriminators).

3. Assign the appropriate clinical priority based on flowchart-guided analysis.

This systematic process minimizes errors and supports accurate prioritization of care.

Priority and Management

It is crucial to differentiate between clinical priority and clinical management. While triage determines the urgency of care, clinical management involves comprehensive understanding of the patient's needs and available resources, which may vary depending on factors such as staffing and bed availability. Proper alignment of these elements ensures streamlined patient flow and equitable resource distribution.

Training and Auditing

Introducing a standardized triage system requires robust training and ongoing evaluation. Practitioners must undergo structured training to develop competence in the methodology, supported by regular audits to ensure consistency and accuracy across departments. Sentinel diagnoses and retrospective reviews serve as benchmarks for evaluating triage performance.

Beyond Emergency Departments

The principles of triage extend beyond emergency departments to other settings, such as primary care and telephone consultations. Modified systems, like the Manchester Triage System (MTS), can be adapted to these contexts. Additionally, triage data can inform dynamic patient monitoring through tools like Early Warning Scores and systems such as the "Manchester Monitor."

Summary

Triage is an indispensable component of emergency care, enabling the prioritization of patients when clinical demand exceeds capacity. By implementing a standardized, teachable, and auditable methodology, the Manchester Triage System ensures patients receive timely care based on clinical urgency. This system supports the dynamic nature of emergency care, enhances patient outcomes, and provides a framework for managing diverse clinical scenarios efficiently.

Through ongoing training and evaluation, triage continues to evolve as a cornerstone of emergency department operations worldwide.

Chapter 2
The Decision-Making Process and Triage

Introduction

Decision-making is a cornerstone of effective medical and nursing practice. It involves both analytical thought and professional intuition, grounded in a solid foundation of knowledge and clinical skill. While some view decision-making as merely "common sense" or "problem-solving," it is, in reality, a sophisticated process requiring a structured approach. In clinical practice, healthcare professionals must interpret, discriminate, and evaluate the information they gather about patients, followed by critical appraisal of their actions. Without a consistent framework, decisions may become unstructured, unreliable, and potentially unsafe. Thus, decision-making is vital for delivering high-quality patient care.

Triage, a critical nursing function, has undergone significant evolution. Historically, during the 1980s, Blythin's SOAP assessment tool was widely used to structure patient interviews, but it lacked guidance on outcomes, leading to variable and subjective triage decisions. The absence of a standardized methodology often resulted in flawed judgments. To address these shortcomings, a robust framework is essential, providing clinicians with the skills and structure necessary to implement effective and reliable triage practices.

Developing Expertise

The progression of clinical expertise follows a continuum comprising five stages:

1. Novice

2. Advanced Beginner

3. Competent

4. Proficient

5. Expert

As clinicians gain experience, their decision-making skills evolve, becoming increasingly nuanced and effective. The transition along this continuum can be facilitated by a methodologically sound system, providing a foundation for consistent and effective decision-making.

Decision-Making Strategies

Several strategies underpin the decision-making process in clinical settings:

1. Reasoning

Inductive Reasoning: This involves analyzing all available data to consider all possible outcomes. While time-intensive, it is particularly beneficial for less experienced clinicians.

Deductive Reasoning: This strategy involves eliminating irrelevant possibilities while gathering patient information. Often employed by experienced practitioners, it enables rapid and focused decision-making.

2. Pattern Recognition
Pattern recognition is crucial for making quick decisions with limited information, especially during triage. Clinicians identify patterns in a patient's symptoms by comparing them to prior cases, leading to a diagnosis or management plan. Expertise enhances this skill, allowing seasoned professionals to intuitively arrive at

decisions, while novices may require more deliberate problem-solving approaches.

3. Repetitive Hypothesizing

This approach tests diagnostic reasoning by collecting data to confirm or refute hypothesis. Depending on the practitioner's level of expertise, it may involve either inductive or deductive reasoning.

4. Mental Representation

Mental representation simplifies complex situations, enabling clinicians to focus on key aspects of the problem. While helpful in complicated cases, it has limited utility in time-sensitive triage scenarios.

5. Intuition

Intuition, often described as a "gut feeling," is deeply intertwined with expertise. It allows practitioners to make rapid and effective decisions with minimal conscious analysis, drawing from tacit knowledge and past experiences. While challenging to quantify, its value in clinical practice is well-documented.

Decision-Making in Triage

Decision-making, whether simple or complex, follows a structured process encompassing three key phases:

1. Problem Identification
Gathering information from patients, caregivers, or pre-hospital personnel to define the issue clearly. This step often involves using a predefined flow diagram for guidance.

2. Information Gathering and Analysis
Utilizing flow diagrams and structured questions to assess the situation rapidly and

effectively. Pattern recognition plays a critical role in this phase.

3. Evaluation and Selection of Alternatives
Clinicians analyze collected data, often stored mentally in an organized framework. Flow diagrams help structure this process, enabling clinicians to evaluate and prioritize options for action.

4. Implementation
Triage decisions are categorized into specific urgency levels, guiding the appropriate care pathway.

5. Monitoring and Evaluation
Triage is a dynamic process, requiring regular reassessment to ensure the assigned category remains accurate. Tools like the Manchester Monitor enable auditing and provide valuable feedback for system improvements.

Challenges in Adopting New Frameworks

Introducing a standardized triage framework may challenge experienced practitioners accustomed to individualized decision-making methods developed over years of practice. However, this change should be embraced as a refinement, offering a rationale for decisions and creating an auditable system. Such a systematic approach enhances teaching for junior staff, providing them with a clear and reliable structure for clinical decision-making.

The triage methodology presented in this manual is adaptable to various practice settings and is beneficial for healthcare providers across all levels of experience. It represents a significant advancement in decision-making processes, promoting consistency, reliability, and quality in patient care.

Chapter 3
The Triage Method

Introduction

This chapter presents a triage method designed for healthcare practitioners to quickly prioritize patients based on clinical urgency. The system focuses on prioritizing patients based on their presenting symptoms rather than assumptions about diagnosis. This approach is consistent with the recognition that Emergency Departments are primarily driven by the immediate signs and symptoms of patients. The triage process follows five steps, as outlined in Chapter 2:

1. Identify the problem.

2. Gather and analyze relevant information.

3. Evaluate possible alternatives and select the most appropriate action.

4. Implement the selected action.

5. Monitor the process and assess outcomes.

Identifying the Problem

In clinical practice, the primary focus is on the patient's presenting complaint, which often refers to the main symptom or concern identified by the patient or caregiver. The list of common presentations pertinent to triage is as follows:

Abdominal pain (adults and children)

Abscesses and infections

Allergic reactions

Asthma

Back pain

Chest pain

Trauma (e.g., falls, head injury, major trauma)

Mental health concerns

Poisoning and overdose

Shortness of breath

Pregnancy-related issues

Diarrhea and vomiting

Rashes and wounds

This list, developed through extensive discussion, encompasses most scenarios encountered in Emergency Departments. It has been slightly updated in this edition, incorporating new categories such as allergies and palpitations, while expanding on facial problems and refining existing classifications like diarrhea and vomiting. The list is broadly categorized into illness, injury, child-specific issues, unusual behavior, and major incidents.

The triage process begins by selecting the appropriate presentation from the list. After this, the practitioner is directed to a corresponding flowchart that includes discriminators—factors used to assess clinical priority. Special care has been taken to ensure these flowcharts are consistent, as some complaints may correspond to multiple charts. For example, a patient presenting with a stiff neck and headache may be categorized under several charts but assigned the same priority.

Gathering and Analyzing Information

Once the correct presentation flowchart is selected, the practitioner must gather and evaluate relevant information to determine the appropriate clinical priority. Each flowchart includes key discriminators, which are questions that guide the practitioner to assess the severity of the patient's condition. The highest level of priority is determined by the answer to these questions.

Discriminators

Discriminators are factors that differentiate between patients and help allocate them to one of five clinical priority categories. These can be general or specific. General discriminators apply to all patients and are found frequently across various charts. Specific discriminators, on the other hand, are tied to particular conditions or presentations.

For instance, severe pain is a general discriminator that appears across many charts, whereas cardiac pain or pleuritic pain are specific to certain conditions. A clear understanding of both general and specific discriminators is essential for accurate triage.

General Discriminators

1. Life Threat: Identifies situations where a patient's life is at risk. This includes compromised airway, breathing difficulties, or cardiac arrest.

2. Hemorrhage: Includes exsanguinating hemorrhage (life-threatening bleeding), major hemorrhage (uncontrolled), and minor hemorrhage (controlled but ongoing).

3. Pain: Severe or moderate pain levels are key to determining triage priority. Severe pain, often described as "the worst pain ever," demands immediate attention, while moderate pain may be addressed after more urgent cases.

4. Conscious Level: Any change in consciousness—whether unconsciousness, altered responsiveness, or confusion—demands prompt triage. This includes cases of patients intoxicated by drugs or alcohol, which should be treated with the same urgency as other causes of altered consciousness.

5. Temperature: Extreme body temperatures (both high and low) signal critical conditions. A patient with a very high temperature (over 41°C) or cold temperature (below 35°C) is considered in immediate need of care.

6. Acuteness: The onset of symptoms plays a role in prioritizing care. Sudden or acute

conditions that began recently (within hours or days) require quicker response compared to chronic issues. However, this does not imply that patients with long-standing conditions should experience extended wait times.

Secondary Triage

In high-volume departments, it may not be feasible to complete all assessments during the initial triage encounter. In these cases, secondary assessments should be carried out by a receiving nurse. These additional assessments provide more detailed information and help refine the clinical priority based on evolving symptoms.

Triage Activity Assessment

1. Greeting the Patient: The assessment process begins the moment the patient enters the triage area. Observing their

appearance as they approach provides valuable insight into their condition. Key visual signs to assess include:

Mobility level: Can the patient walk unaided, or are they struggling to move?

Obvious injuries: Are there any visible wounds or signs of trauma?

Patient's age: Age can be a significant factor in determining the urgency of care needed.

2. Patient History: The triage process involves asking the patient to explain the reason for their visit to the emergency department. This step gathers a succinct, subjective history that reveals their injury, illness, or any other health-related issue. The goal is to quickly identify the nature of the problem.

3. Presenting Complaint: The presenting complaint, or the main reason for the patient's visit, is derived from their history. Understanding the complaint enables the nurse to determine which triage flow chart to follow to assess the situation further.

4. Focused Questions (Interview): This phase highlights the triage practitioner's expertise. It involves utilizing anatomical knowledge, recognizing patterns in symptoms, and responding appropriately to life-threatening situations. Focused questions allow for a more in-depth understanding of the issue, such as:

The duration of symptoms

The mechanism of injury

Current medications These questions are guided by the discriminators in the selected presentation flow chart.

5. Physical Examination and Assessment of Physical Parameters: If necessary, physical assessment may include:

Location of injuries: Identifying the exact sites of injury or concern.

Baseline observations: Such as pulse, temperature, or detailed data like pulse oximetry or visual acuity.

6. Pain Assessment: Pain assessment is a critical part of the Manchester Triage System (MTS). Both subjective pain scores (as reported by the patient) and objective scores (as assessed by the triage practitioner) are recorded. It's important to document the rationale behind any discrepancies between the two scores.

7. Priority/Plan of Care: Once the assessment is complete, a clinical priority is assigned based on the highest discriminator relevant to the patient's condition. The triage

practitioner should also outline any immediate care that the patient may need based on the assessment findings.

8. Documentation: Accurate and relevant documentation is crucial in triage. All recorded information should be clear, concise, and directly related to the presenting issue. If a computerized triage system is used, it is important for the practitioner to maintain focus on the patient rather than the screen or keyboard. Documentation should include:

Allergies

Current medications

Relevant medical history

First aid measures applied at triage

Observations taken during triage

Medications given (e.g., analgesia)

The practitioner's legible signature.

9. Reassessment: It is essential to document when reassessment is necessary, particularly if pain relief (analgesia) has been administered. This ensures ongoing evaluation of the patient's condition and that care is adjusted as needed.

10. Monitoring and Evaluation: The clinical priority of a patient can change over time, and as such, triage must be a dynamic process. The method described allows for quick, reliable evaluations by trained personnel, which is especially useful for re-assessing clinical priority throughout the patient's stay in the emergency department. Regular nursing assessments can identify changes in the patient's condition, ensuring that any shift in clinical priority is promptly addressed. This process facilitates continuous monitoring of the patient's

condition and provides a clear guide for decision-making.

The triage methodology ensures that patient assessment is conducted swiftly and accurately, enabling healthcare providers to make informed decisions on the urgency of care required.

Chapter 4
Pain Assessment as Part of the Triage Process

Introduction

Pain is a significant aspect of patient care in the Emergency Department (ED). Available evidence suggests that pain is a central concern for patients, yet it is often poorly assessed and inadequately managed, leading to suboptimal outcomes (termed oligoanalgesia). Addressing pain effectively is crucial for several reasons:

1. Prevalence of Pain: A large proportion of ED patients present with some degree of pain.

2. Influence on Triage: The severity of pain influences the urgency of care.

3. Patient Satisfaction: Proper pain management is closely tied to patient satisfaction.

4. Behavioral Impact: Unmanaged pain can cause agitation or aggression in patients.

5. Staff Well-being: Painful patient experiences create stress for healthcare staff.

6. Patient Expectations: Patients anticipate that their pain will be promptly and effectively addressed.

Incorporating pain assessment into the triage process offers several advantages. It facilitates early pain management, potentially lowering patient priority levels, which optimizes resource allocation. Additionally, addressing pain reduces anxiety, improves communication, and ensures timely analgesia at the point of triage.

Pain Assessment Process in Triage

Pain assessment is a core component of triage, especially within structured systems like the Manchester Triage System. This approach acknowledges pain's significance and has intentionally increased the priority for some patients to counter historically poor pain management practices.

For pain assessments to be effective, they must be valid, reproducible, and performed by trained triage practitioners. Over-reliance on subjective patient reporting or isolated assessments by staff can compromise the accuracy of triage decisions.

Challenges of Pain Assessment in Emergency Settings

Pain assessment in the ED is complex due to several factors:

Subjectivity: Patients may exaggerate or understate pain based on perceived benefits or fears.

Traditional Practices: Historical norms may bias practitioners (e.g., fractures are prioritized for analgesia, while abdominal pain might be delayed for diagnostic clarity).

Misinterpretation of Pain Scales: Patients may manipulate scores to expedite care.

Pain Assessment Tools

Formal tools are increasingly used in EDs, although many were originally designed for postoperative or chronic pain patients. Common pain assessment tools include:

1. Verbal Descriptor Scales: Patients select descriptors (e.g., "None," "Moderate," "Severe") that correlate with pain intensity.

Advantages: Quick, easy to use, reliable in certain settings.

Disadvantages: Limited by language barriers and subjective interpretation.

2. Visual Analogue Scales (VAS): Patients mark their pain intensity on a line anchored by "No Pain" and "Worst Pain Possible."

Advantages: Sensitive, quick to use, and reliable when applied correctly.

Disadvantages: Challenging for certain populations (e.g., elderly, low literacy).

3. Pain Behavior Tools: Assess behavioral and physiological indicators of pain (e.g., facial expressions, verbal responses).

Advantages: Useful for non-verbal or cognitively impaired patients.

Disadvantages: Time-consuming, complex to interpret, and may confound pain with other stressors.

The Ideal Pain Assessment Tool

An effective tool in the ED should be simple, rapid, reliable, and validated. It should integrate patient-reported and observer-measured data.

The Pain Ruler exemplifies a versatile assessment tool for the ED:

Combines verbal descriptors and visual analogues.

Measures pain intensity and its impact on normal functioning.

Facilitates triage by producing quick, documentable scores.

Encourages patient-nurse dialogue, demonstrating empathy and commitment to pain relief.

Supplementary tools like a Faces Scale are helpful for assessing pain in children.

Key Considerations in Triage Pain Assessment

1. Age:

Children: Often exaggerate pain due to anxiety and catastrophic thinking.

Elderly: May under report pain due to tolerance or coping mechanisms.

Assessment Tips: Understand age-related perceptions and adapt accordingly.

2. Previous Pain Experience:

Patients compare current pain with past episodes, influencing their perception.

Assessment Tips: Explore prior pain management experiences and outcomes.

3. Cultural Influences:

Cultural and social norms shape pain expression. Practitioners must acknowledge their biases when interpreting patient behavior.

Assessment Tips: Recognize the influence of cultural backgrounds on pain reporting.

4. Anxiety:

High anxiety amplifies pain perception.

Assessment Tips: Address underlying concerns to alleviate anxiety and reduce perceived pain.

5. Impact on Daily Activities:

Pain disrupts physical, emotional, and social functioning.

Assessment Tips: Assess how pain affects activities like eating, sleeping, or working to gauge its severity.

6. Special Populations:

Patients with cognitive impairments, language barriers, or distress may require alternative assessment methods.

Assessment Tips: Tailor tools and approaches to individual patient needs.

Conclusion

Pain assessment during triage is essential for delivering timely and effective care in the ED. While constraints such as time and variability in patient presentation pose challenges, skilled assessments guided by validated tools can significantly improve outcomes. Recognizing the subjective and multifaceted nature of pain ensures a more empathetic and comprehensive approach to emergency care.

Chapter 5
Patient Management, Triage, and the Role of the Triage Nurse

Introduction

Effective triage in emergency settings is pivotal for patient care. This process involves distinguishing absolute clinical priorities, as outlined in this guide, from relative priorities within and across triage categories. The fundamental steps of triage are straightforward: patients are classified into categories based on urgency and attended to in sequence of priority and arrival time. However, numerous factors beyond clinical urgency can influence patient management within the Emergency Department (ED). This chapter explores these factors, emphasizing their significance in optimizing departmental operations and enhancing patient care outcomes. Recognizing and addressing these considerations is crucial to maintaining a functional ED and ensuring high-quality care.

Patient-Specific Considerations

Children

Managing pediatric patients requires a tailored approach, particularly in EDs without dedicated pediatric services. These patients often arrive accompanied by caregivers—parents, relatives, or professionals—and possibly siblings or friends. Children's short attention spans, combined with their propensity to experience boredom, fear, and fatigue, can lead to distress and agitation, complicating subsequent care.

Providing distractions like play areas and snacks (where appropriate) can help.

Policies for late-night arrivals, such as prioritizing tired children for early assessment, can prevent challenges in care delivery.

Elderly Patients

Older adults face unique challenges in the ED:

Reduced mobility and increased discomfort may hinder their ability to navigate the facility.

Routine disruptions can cause confusion and anxiety.

They are at higher risk of tissue damage from prolonged immobility and may require more frequent nursing attention.

Practitioners must account for potential memory issues and continence problems, ensuring adequate and respectful care.

Patients with Disabilities or Learning Difficulties

Patients with sensory impairments or cognitive challenges often struggle in unfamiliar environments like the ED.

Effective communication and prioritization can alleviate their distress.

Addressing their needs promptly ensures they receive equitable care without undue delays.

Aggressive or Abusive Patients

Disruptive behavior, often stemming from frustration, can affect the entire waiting area.

Strategies include isolating such patients in individual rooms or expediting their care to minimize disruptions.

Persistent issues may necessitate security or law enforcement involvement to ensure safety.

Patients Under the Influence of Alcohol

Alcohol-intoxicated individuals are challenging to evaluate due to altered consciousness and pain perception.

Regular reassessment is critical to identify hidden or evolving medical conditions.

Disruptive patients should be managed following guidelines for aggressive behavior.

Frequent Visitors (Regulars)

Regular ED users may be at higher risk for underlying health issues despite their frequent presentations.

Each visit should be treated independently, with proper evaluation to avoid missing critical diagnoses.

Re-Attending Patients

Patients returning to the ED often do so because of unresolved issues or complications.

Their triage category should reflect their current symptoms rather than their initial visit's assessment.

In some cases, a review by senior clinicians or referral to a follow-up clinic may be appropriate.

Clinic Patients and Referrals

Patients attending scheduled clinics or referred by other agencies, such as primary care physicians or social services, must be triaged like any other ED patient.

Clear communication with referral teams ensures timely care for these patients.

Immediate interventions, such as analgesia or diagnostic tests, may streamline their ED experience.

Departmental Dynamics

Overcrowding and Resource Management

Emergency departments often face surges in patient volume or staff shortages, impacting workflow.

Accurate triage is essential for prioritizing care during such periods.

Adjustments like addressing quick cases first or prioritizing children late at night can help manage workload effectively.

Fast-Tracking and Streaming

Streaming involves categorizing patients into specific care pathways managed by dedicated staff, improving efficiency. Fast-tracking applies a similar principle, focusing on patients with minor injuries or conditions.

The Manchester Triage System facilitates these processes, aligning resources with patient needs.

Managing Quiet Periods

During quieter times, maintaining workflow momentum is essential to prevent unnecessary delays and ensure timely care.

Role of the Triage Nurse

Key Responsibilities

The triage nurse plays a critical role in ensuring accurate patient prioritization.

Rapid decision-making and delegation of non-urgent tasks are crucial.

Clear communication with patients and their caregivers alleviates anxiety and sets expectations.

First Aid and Pain Management

Providing immediate interventions, such as applying dressings or administering analgesics, improves patient comfort and prevents further complications.

Health Promotion

If time permits, triage nurses can offer brief health advice or distribute educational materials, enhancing preventive care.

Dynamic Patient Reassessment

Triage is an ongoing process. Patients in the waiting room require periodic reassessment, particularly after interventions like pain management or significant delays.

Optimizing ED Flow

Patient Placement

Strategic placement of patients within the ED enhances comfort and care delivery:

Patients in pain, with bleeding, or at the extremes of age benefit from quiet, dedicated spaces.

Those requiring specific examinations should be directed to appropriate areas.

Waiting Room Management

Continuous observation and communication are essential in managing the waiting room effectively.

Regular updates on waiting times and prompt identification of deteriorating patients ensure safety and satisfaction.

This chapter emphasizes the importance of a comprehensive, patient-centered approach to triage and patient management in the ED. By addressing both clinical and non-clinical factors, healthcare providers can deliver efficient, equitable, and high-quality care, even in challenging environments.

Chapter 6
Auditing the Triage Process

Introduction

In November 1994, the Manchester Triage Group (MTG) established a clear goal: to ensure a robust audit methodology. This decision was critical, as the Manchester Triage System (MTS) was designed to reduce inconsistencies in the triage process. To achieve this goal, a quality management procedure like auditing was deemed essential. Since triage is fundamental to clinical risk management, any compromise in its quality could have significant repercussions.

The Manchester Triage System is highly auditable due to its structured progression—from presenting condition to discriminator to assigned priority. This process allows trained auditors to easily evaluate the accuracy and consistency of triage decisions. Research indicates that even untrained assessors demonstrate reasonable agreement in their evaluations, while trained professionals achieve a high level of consistency.

In addition to assessing triage accuracy, audits can identify issues such as incomplete documentation or misuse of terminology, as practitioners under pressure may invent new discriminators. This chapter outlines a systematic audit approach for the Manchester Triage System and presents insights from audits conducted globally.

Audit Methodology

The cornerstone of a robust audit system lies in continuously evaluating the accuracy of triage practitioners. This process incorporates reflective practices and, where necessary, additional training to improve performance. The steps below outline a structured approach to auditing triage activity:

1. Identification of Practitioners: All triage practitioners are cataloged.

2. Compilation of Episodes: Every triage episode is recorded and linked to individual practitioners.

3. Random Sampling: A minimum of 2% of episodes per practitioner (at least 10 episodes) is randomly selected for review.

4. Assessment by Senior Practitioners: Episodes are reviewed by experienced senior triage practitioners.

5. Evaluation Metrics:

Completeness: Determined as a proportion of episodes with all required steps completed.

Accuracy: Calculated as a proportion of episodes where the correct presentation, discriminator, and priority were selected.

6. Feedback: Practitioners receive feedback on incomplete episodes, overall accuracy, and any causes of inaccuracy.

To ensure consistency, 10% of audited episodes are independently reviewed by a second senior practitioner, and discrepancies are resolved through discussion. While time-intensive, continuous audits provide a reliable measure of triage standards. During initial implementation, monthly audits are recommended. Even in high-volume settings managing 100,000 patients annually, only about 2,000 cases (160 per month) need auditing. Over time, the frequency can be reduced to every three to six months.

Key Criteria for Assessment

A comprehensive audit tool should evaluate the following:

Correct use of presentation flowcharts.

Accurate recording of specific discriminators.

Documentation of pain scores.

Assignment of appropriate triage categories based on patient presentation.

Legibility and signature of triage records.

Re-triaging where necessary.

These elements are summarized in a flow diagram that calculates accuracy and completeness percentages, with the following targets:

0% incomplete episodes.

95% accuracy.

95% inter-assessor agreement.

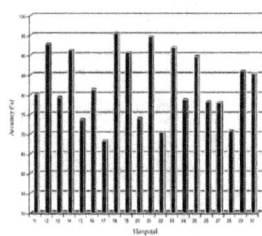

Completeness and Accuracy Defined

Completeness:

An episode is complete when all steps necessary to reach a conclusion are undertaken. This includes ruling out all higher-priority discriminators. For example, if SaO2 is listed as a discriminator, failure to record a result would render the episode incomplete. Pain scores are the most frequently omitted data point.

Accuracy:

An accurate episode is one where the selected presentation and discriminator align with the patient's condition. The system's flexibility permits valid alternatives, but this judgment requires an experienced auditor.

Practical Impact of Audits

Audits directly improve triage documentation and accuracy. For example, omitting pain scores or physiological measurements like peak expiratory flow rate (PEFR) or temperature will result in episodes being marked as incomplete. Feedback encourages better compliance, with measurable improvements in record-keeping observed early in the auditing process.

Case Studies and Findings

Regional Audit in England:

A study across a health region audited 100 triage episodes per center. Each episode was reviewed by two senior practitioners, with 10% undergoing further independent review. Accuracy varied between 68% and 95%, reflecting differences in case mix and demonstrating that computer-assisted triage systems enhanced accuracy.

National Audit in Portugal:

Portugal implemented the MTS nationally in 2001, mandating continuous audits. Results reported to the Portuguese Triage Group (GPT) showed high accuracy rates. Contrary to concerns about delays, the audits revealed that triage interventions typically took 30–60 seconds. Delays in emergency department throughput were attributed to tasks unrelated to triage.

Conclusion

Auditing the triage process is an essential quality assurance measure that enhances the reliability and efficiency of the Manchester Triage System. By focusing on accuracy and completeness, regular audits drive improvements in documentation, decision-making, and patient outcomes. Global case studies underscore the value of robust audit methodologies in achieving consistent and high-quality triage practices.

CHAPTER 7
Telephone Triage

Introduction

The concept of formalized telephone triage originated in the United States and was later adopted in the United Kingdom. By 1991, telephone triage was recognized as a valuable tool in emergency settings across the UK. This system offers numerous benefits, such as reducing unnecessary emergency department (ED) visits through explanations and self-care advice, redirecting patients to appropriate services, identifying critical issues before arrival, improving cost efficiency, and empowering patients with informed decision-making.

Historically, providing advice over the telephone has been an integral part of nursing practice, although it was not always recognized as a specialized function. Initial studies revealed significant gaps in early telephone-based assessments, which were often subjective, poorly structured, and conducted by untrained individuals. Decisions were frequently made without gathering comprehensive information. Recommendations from these studies emphasized the importance of trained advisors, structured protocols, and proper documentation to ensure informed and safe decision-making. When implemented effectively, telephone triage has proven to be a reliable and safe prioritization method, paving the way for innovations such as NHS Direct, a telephone advice and helpline service in the UK.

The distinction between telephone advice and telephone triage lies in the formalization of the decision-making process. Telephone triage involves assessing clinical priority and assigning urgency levels for medical evaluation and care based on established protocols.

Telephone Triage Methodology

Effective triage, whether face-to-face or via telephone, focuses on assessing clinical priority based on symptoms rather than diagnosis. Telephone triage methodology, derived from the Manchester Triage Group's face-to-face model, simplifies decision-making into three possible outcomes:

1. Immediate and urgent care required (Medicine Now)

2. Care needed within a few hours (Medicine Soon)

3. Care can be delayed (Medicine Later)

Patients in the "Medicine Now" category should immediately access emergency services, such as an ambulance or ED. For patients in the "Medicine Soon" category, care delivery depends on the triage setting. For instance, ED-based triage might recommend urgent self-transport, whereas primary care might direct the patient to the nearest clinic for same-day evaluation. "Medicine Later" patients can often manage symptoms at home or seek care at their convenience. Access to accurate local service information, such as emergency dental services, after-hours pharmacies, and primary care contacts, is crucial for effective telephone triage.

Decision-Making Process

The telephone triage process begins with gathering key information from the caller about the nature of the problem. This helps the practitioner select the appropriate flowchart for further questioning. The decision-making process involves systematically assessing potential serious conditions first, progressing to less critical possibilities.

For example, back pain might be evaluated based on discriminators such as:

Airway compromise

Inadequate breathing

Recent trauma

Neurological deficits

The practitioner determines the priority level by assessing whether the patient's symptoms meet criteria for each discriminator. Discriminator definitions and specific questions tailored to the telephone setting are essential to account for the remote nature of assessments. For instance:

Discriminator	Questions	Definition
Acute onset after injury	Did this start after a fall or trauma?	Symptoms immediately following a traumatic event
Shortness of breath	Has this come on suddenly? Is it worse than normal?	Sudden or severe breathing difficulty
Cardiac pain	Where is the pain? Does it radiate to your arm or neck?	Classic breathing chest pain, possibly radiating and associated with nausea/sweating

Interim Advice

Because the patient is not physically present, interim advice may be necessary to stabilize their condition until medical help arrives. Examples include:

Seizures: Place the patient in the recovery position, loosen clothing, and avoid inserting objects into their mouth.

High fever in children: Remove excess clothing and administer age-appropriate doses of paracetamol.

Poison ingestion: Avoid inducing vomiting; provide sips of cold water for burning sensations in the mouth.

Interim advice must be tailored to the specific discriminator and situation, ensuring safety until appropriate care is available.

Pain Assessment

Pain evaluation is integral to triage but presents unique challenges in telephone settings. Observation is impossible, and patients may struggle to articulate pain levels accurately. Within telephone triage systems, severe pain is a critical discriminator that automatically places the patient in the "Medicine Now" category. Other prioritization decisions rely on additional clinical information obtained during questioning.

The Role of the Telephone Triage Practitioner

Telephone triage requires experienced practitioners with advanced clinical knowledge and refined questioning skills. Unlike face-to-face triage, telephone assessments rely entirely on verbal communication, requiring practitioners to extract accurate information efficiently from potentially distressed callers.

Protocols and flowcharts support the decision-making process, but clinical judgment remains paramount. Proper training and continuous auditing of systems ensure consistent and effective use of telephone triage methodologies.

Conclusion

Telephone triage offers a structured, auditable approach to prioritizing patients in emergency care settings. By adhering to established protocols and leveraging skilled practitioners, this methodology ensures safe, efficient, and patient-centered care, even in remote interactions.

Chapter 8
Beyond Prioritization

The Triage System was initially created as a comprehensive and auditable clinical risk management tool aimed at determining the priority of patient care based on clinical urgency. However, as this book has previously noted, the application of the Triage System extends beyond the prioritization of patients. This chapter highlights two additional utilities of Triage System: dynamic patient monitoring and decision-making through the presentation-priority matrix.

Dynamic Monitoring:

Triage is an ongoing process requiring periodic reassessment of patients while they await treatment. This ensures any changes in a patient's condition are promptly identified, allowing for necessary adjustments in their triage category. Such monitoring remains essential even after the initial clinical consultation, as timely detection of deterioration is critical for initiating appropriate reassessments and interventions.

In some hospital settings, monitoring is performed effectively using an "early warning score" system. However, in emergency departments, implementing this approach often requires clinicians to adapt to new tools. Instead, the existing discriminators within the Triage System—particularly those addressing airway, breathing, and circulation (ABC) threats—offer a practical framework for ongoing assessment.

Key Discriminators and Actions:

Red Discriminator: Signals immediate reassessment.

Orange Discriminator: Requires action within 10 minutes.

Yellow Discriminator: Needs intervention within 60 minutes.

This monitoring strategy leverages a tool familiar to nursing staff, enhancing efficiency and ensuring rapid responses to changes in patient conditions.

Presentation-Priority Matrix Mapping

As emergency care evolves, concepts like "emergency care villages" and multiple access points are replacing traditional notions of an "inappropriate patient." Clinicians now need tools that align patient needs with the most appropriate care settings.

The MTS Presentation-Priority Matrix captures triage outcomes to guide decisions on patient disposition. Each MTS presentation (e.g., chest pain, limb injury) is paired with a priority level (e.g., urgent, very urgent), forming a "presentation-priority complex." This matrix facilitates matching patients with suitable care areas, such as minor injury units, resuscitation rooms, or primary care centers.

Matrix Utilization:

1. Defined Dispositions:

Example: A patient with a limb injury at standard priority might be directed to a minor injuries unit.

Critical Case: A patient with chest pain marked as very urgent is best managed in the resuscitation area.

2. Grey Areas: Some conditions may fit multiple care settings, requiring clinician judgment to determine the best option based on service availability and patient needs.

3. Local Variability: The matrix is adaptable to regional differences in emergency care provisions, such as the presence or absence of specialized units (e.g., ophthalmic or psychiatric services).

Future Implications:

Accurate triage is vital to the matrix's success, as disposition decisions heavily rely on the precision of initial assessments. The matrix also promotes dialogue about optimizing local emergency services and resource allocation.

Extended Functions of Triage Consultations

In addition to prioritization, triage practitioners may engage in several extended functions, including:

Pain Management: Administering analgesics to alleviate discomfort.

Direct Referrals: Sending patients for immediate imaging, such as X-rays.

Pathway Initiation: Referring patients to self-care, pharmacies, general practitioners, or in-patient specialties based on predefined pathways.

Benefits of Extended Triage:

1. Enhanced Patient Experience: Early pain relief reduces distress.

2. Streamlined Processes: Pre-ordered investigations (e.g., X-rays) can minimize delays in definitive care.

3. Efficient Resource Use: Direct referrals optimize resource allocation and avoid unnecessary delays.

Challenges and Solutions:

Increased Consultation Times: Extended assessments may lead to delays in triage.

Solution: Employ multiple triage practitioners simultaneously to maintain efficiency.

Training Needs: Additional education is required for nurses to confidently manage expanded responsibilities.

Conclusion

The Manchester Triage System has proven its value beyond patient prioritization, offering tools for real-time monitoring and guiding disposition decisions. While these extended applications improve patient care and system efficiency, their implementation must be evidence-based and supported by adequate resources and training.

Differentiation Glossary

Abdominal Pain: Pain experienced in the abdomen. If associated with back pain, it may indicate an abdominal aortic aneurysm. If associated with pelvic vaginal bleeding, it could suggest an ectopic pregnancy or miscarriage.

Abnormal Pulse: A pulse rate below 60 beats per minute (bradycardia), above 100 beats per minute (tachycardia), or an irregular rhythm. Definitions for bradycardia and tachycardia should be adjusted for pediatric patients.

Abrupt Onset: Symptoms occurring rapidly, within seconds or minutes, and possibly disrupting sleep.

Acute Chemical Eye Injury: Exposure to a substance within the last 24 hours causing stinging, burning, or diminished vision in the eye, suggesting a chemical injury.

Acute Complete Loss of Vision: Sudden loss of vision in one or both eyes that has not returned to normal within 24 hours.

Acute Neurological Deficit: Any sudden loss of neurological function within the last 24 hours, which may include altered sensation, limb weakness (either transient or permanent), or changes in bladder or bowel control.

Acute Onset After Injury: Onset of symptoms within 24 hours following a physical injury.

Acutely Avulsed Tooth: A tooth that has been completely knocked out within the last 24 hours.

Acutely Short of Breath: Sudden onset of shortness of breath or a significant worsening of chronic shortness of breath.

Age Less Than 25 Years: Individuals who are 25 years old or younger.

Airway Compromise: A compromised airway occurs when it cannot be kept open, or when protective reflexes (to prevent inhalation) are lost. This may result in partial or total obstruction, indicated by snoring or bubbling sounds during breathing.

Altered Blood: Blood that appears darker than fresh blood, often with a more pronounced odor, resembling melena.

Altered Conscious Level: A reduced level of awareness, where the patient may only respond to voice or pain, or is unresponsive.

Altered Conscious Level Not Attributable to Alcohol: A patient who is not fully alert, with a history of alcohol consumption, where no other cause of reduced consciousness is evident.

Altered Conscious Level Wholly Attributable to Alcohol: A patient who is not fully alert, with a clear history of alcohol consumption, and no other cause of reduced consciousness can be identified.

Altered Facial Sensation: Any change in sensation on the face.

Atypical Behaviour: Children exhibiting unusual behavior in a given situation, often described as fractious or out of sorts by their caregivers.

Auricular Haematoma: A swollen collection of blood in the outer ear, typically resulting from trauma.

Black Stool: Stool that appears black in color, typically indicative of gastrointestinal bleeding.

Bleeding Disorder: A congenital or acquired condition that affects blood clotting and causes abnormal bleeding.

Breathing After Airway Opening: In major incidents, the presence of breathing after a simple airway opening maneuver allows for respiratory rate measurement. Absence of breathing after airway opening suggests death.

Capillary Refill Time: The time it takes for nail bed capillaries to refill after being compressed for 5 seconds. A normal time is under 2 seconds. This sign is less reliable if the patient is cold.

Capillary Refill Time Abnormal: In major incidents, patients with prolonged capillary refill time (greater than 2 seconds) are categorized as high priority (RED).

Cardiac Pain: A severe, dull, "gripping" chest pain that may radiate to the left arm or neck, often associated with sweating and nausea.

Chemical Injury: Exposure to any substance that causes stinging, burning, or reduced vision, or other symptoms, which could result in a chemical injury.

Chest Infection: Typically characterized by cough and sputum production, which is often purulent (green or yellow).

Chest Injury: Any injury affecting the area between the clavicles and the lowest rib. Injury to the lower chest may also affect abdominal organs.

Cold: When the skin feels cold, the patient is considered clinically cold. Core temperature should be taken as soon as possible. A core temperature below 35°C is considered cold.

Colicky Pain: Pain that occurs in waves. Renal colic, for instance, usually presents with intermittent pain over 20-minute intervals.

Critical Skin: A fracture or dislocation may cause bone fragments or ends to press against the skin, risking the skin's viability. This is characterized by white, tense skin.

Currently Fitting: A patient actively experiencing a tonic-clonic seizure or partial seizures.

Current Palpitation: A sensation of the heart racing or fluttering, still ongoing.

Deformity: Refers to abnormal angulation or rotation, which is always subjective.

Diplopia: Double vision that resolves when one eye is closed.

Direct Trauma to the Back: Any trauma involving the back, such as falling and landing on the feet, bending, or twisting motions.

Direct Trauma to the Neck: Any trauma to the neck, including loading (such as an object falling on the head) or bending/twisting movements.

Discharge: In cases of sexually transmitted infection, any abnormal discharge from the penis or vagina is significant.

Disruptive: Behavior that interferes with the functioning of the department, often threatening in nature.

Distal Vascular Compromise: Characterized by pallor, coldness, altered sensation, pain, and possibly absent pulses distal to the injury site.

Distressed by Pain: A child showing distress and inconsolability due to pain.

Drooling: Saliva running from the mouth due to an inability to swallow.

Dysuria: Pain or discomfort during urination, often described as stinging or burning.

Electrical Injury: Any injury caused by electric current, whether from alternating or direct current, and from natural or artificial sources.

Exhaustion: Patients showing reduced effort in breathing, despite continuing respiratory insufficiency, often a pre terminal sign.

Exsanguinating Haemorrhage: A severe hemorrhage occurring at such a rapid rate that death is imminent unless stopped.

Externalisation of Organs: The protrusion or herniation of internal organs outside the body.

Eye Injury: Any physical trauma to the eye.

Facial Oedema: Generalized swelling around the face, including the lips.

Facial Swelling: Swelling around the face, which may be localized or diffuse.

Fails to React to Parents: The patient does not respond to the presence or voice of a parent, indicating a possible abnormal reaction or lack of recognition.

Floppy: A child described as having reduced muscle tone, often resulting in a limp or head lolling.

Focal or Progressive Loss of Function: Loss of function affecting a specific body part, or worsening over time.

Foreign Body Sensation: The feeling of something in the eye, often described as grittiness or scraping.

Frank Haematuria: The presence of visible blood in the urine.

Fresh Blood: Blood that appears unaltered and can be easily identified by the patient and caregivers.

Generalised Rash: A rash that may be erythematous or urticarial in nature.

Gross Deformity: Abnormal, exaggerated angulation or rotation, typically subjective.

Headache: Pain around the head that is not localized to any specific anatomical structure.

Head Injury: Any trauma to the head.

Heavy PV Blood Loss: Excessive vaginal bleeding, often indicated by large clots or constant flow.

High Blood Pressure: A history or current measurement of elevated blood pressure.

High Lethality: The potential of a substance to cause significant harm, including possible death. In cases of doubt, assume high risk.

High Risk of Harm to Others: When there is a potential for harm to others, indicated by tense posture, threatening speech, or restless behavior. If weapons or potential victims are present, or if self-control is lost, the risk should be considered high.

High Risk of Self-Harm: Assessment of self-harm risk based on patient behavior.

Those with a history of self-harm or actively attempting harm are at higher risk.

History of Acutely Vomiting Blood: Vomiting of fresh or altered blood (e.g., coffee ground appearance) within the last 24 hours.

History of Fitting: Any observed or reported seizures during the current illness or following trauma.

History of Head Injury: A history of recent trauma to the head, typically reported by the patient or a reliable witness if the patient is unconscious.

History of Overdose or Poisoning: Information that may be reported by others or inferred from missing medications or signs of poisoning.

History of Recent Foreign Travel: Travel to a foreign country within the past 2 weeks.

History of Trauma: A history of recent physical injury.

History of Unconsciousness: A reliable witness may confirm whether the patient was unconscious and the duration. If no witness is available, the patient should be assumed unconscious if they cannot recall the event.

Moderate Pain: Pain that is tolerable yet intense. For further evaluation, refer to the section on pain assessment.

Moderate Risk of Harm to Others: The potential risk to others can be assessed by observing the patient's posture (tense or clenched), speech (loud or threatening language), and motor behavior (restlessness or pacing). If any indication of harm exists, a moderate risk should be assumed.

Moderate Risk of Self-Harm: The likelihood of self-harm can be gauged by considering the patient's behavior. Those without a history of self-harm but who express a desire to harm themselves, or show no active intent to harm, are categorized as at moderate risk.

New Neurological Deficit: Any loss of neurological function, including altered or lost sensation, limb weakness (either temporary or permanent), and changes in bladder or bowel function.

No Improvement with Asthma Medications: Failure to show improvement despite the use of prescribed bronchodilators, either by a GP or paramedic, is a critical factor in assessing asthma management.

Non-Blanching Rash: A rash that remains red when pressure is applied, and does not change color (blanch). Often tested using a glass tumbler to apply pressure to observe any color change.

Normal Menstruation: Menstrual blood loss and associated pain occurring within the expected timeframe and duration.

Not Distractible: Children in distress, who are unable to be distracted by conversation or play, are considered to fulfill this criterion.

Not Feeding: Children who are unwilling to consume food or liquid (as appropriate). This may also apply to children who vomit immediately after eating.

Not Passing Urine: Inability to pass urine. This can be difficult to assess in children or the elderly, and it may be helpful to monitor the frequency of nappies or pads used.

Oedema of the Tongue: Swelling of the tongue, regardless of the severity.

Open Fracture: Fractures that are associated with a wound may indicate an open fracture. If there is any doubt about the presence of a wound communicating with the fracture, it should be considered open.

Pain on Joint Movement: Pain caused by either active movement (patient) or passive movement (examiner) of a joint.

Pain Radiating to the Back: Pain that extends to the back, either intermittently or persistently.

Passing Fresh or Altered Blood per Rectum (PR): Massive gastrointestinal bleeding typically results in dark red blood being passed via the rectum. As the blood moves through the GI tract, it becomes darker, potentially appearing as melena.

PEFR <33% Predicted: The peak expiratory flow rate (PEFR) predicted for the patient, based on their age and sex. If the measured

PEFR is less than 33% of the predicted value, this criterion is met.

PEFR <50% Predicted: If the measured PEFR is less than 50% of the predicted value based on age and sex, this criterion is met.

Penetrating Eye Injury: An injury where the eye globe has been penetrated by a foreign object.

Penetrating Trauma: Any traumatic event that involves a penetrating injury to the body, such as from a knife, bullet, or similar object.

Persistent Vomiting: Continuous vomiting or vomiting episodes that do not have any relief between them

Pleuritic Pain: Sharp, localized chest pain that worsens with breathing, coughing, or sneezing.

Possibly Pregnant: A woman who has missed her period may be considered potentially pregnant. This includes women of childbearing age who are engaging in unprotected sex.

Presenting Fetal Parts: Any part of the fetus, such as the head or limbs, visibly protruding from the vagina (e.g., crowning).

Priapism: A persistent, often painful, erection of the penis.

Prolapsed Umbilical Cord: The umbilical cord slips through the cervix, posing a risk to the fetus.

Prolonged or Uninterrupted Crying: A child crying continuously for two hours or more is classified under this criterion.

Pulse Rate Abnormal: A pulse rate over 120 beats per minute indicates an urgent condition, especially if capillary refill time cannot be measured.

Purpura: A rash caused by small blood vessel hemorrhages beneath the skin. It does not blanch when pressure is applied.

PV Blood Loss: Loss of blood via the vaginal route.

PV Blood Loss and More Than 20 Weeks Pregnant: Any vaginal bleeding in a pregnant woman beyond the 20th week of gestation.

Rapid Onset: Symptoms or condition onset occurring within the past 12 hours.

Recent Hearing Loss: Loss of hearing in one or both ears occurring within the last week.

Recent Injury: Injuries that occurred within the past week.

Recent Mild Itch: An itching sensation that has occurred within the past week.

Recent Mild Pain: Pain experienced within the last week.

Recent Problem: Any medical issue that has arisen in the past week.

Recent Reduced Visual Acuity: Any reduction in corrected visual acuity experienced within the last week.

Recent Signs of Mild Pain: Young children and infants who cannot verbally express pain often show signs of distress, such as crying and changes in behavior.

Redcurrant Stool: A dark red stool commonly associated with intussusception. However, its absence does not rule out this diagnosis.

Red Eye: Any redness in the eye, which may be accompanied by pain or be painless. It can affect part or all of the eye.

Respiratory Rate: Patients whose respiratory rate is abnormally high (over 29) or low (under 10) are classified under red triage.

Responds to Pain: The patient's reaction to painful stimuli, typically applied to the nail bed. Avoid using supraorbital ridge pressure to prevent reflex grimacing in cases of brain death.

Responds to Voice: The patient's reaction to vocal stimuli. It is important not to shout the patient's name unless necessary, as children may fail to respond due to fear.

Retention of Urine: The inability to urinate due to an enlarged bladder, typically a painful condition unless there is altered sensation.

Risk of Continued Contamination: If exposure to chemicals is ongoing or if proper decontamination has not occurred, the patient and healthcare workers may continue to be at risk.

Risk of Harm to Others: The potential for a patient to cause harm to others, evaluated by considering the patient's mental state, posture, and behavior. In case of doubt, assume a high risk.

Risk of Self-Harm: The potential for a patient to attempt self-harm. If uncertain, assume a high risk.

Scalp Haematoma: A raised bruised area on the scalp, often found below the hairline at the forehead.

Scrotal Cellulitis: Swelling and redness around the scrotum.

Scrotal Gangrene: Necrosis of the skin around the scrotum, which may appear black or as a full-thickness burn. Early gangrene may not be black but could resemble burn tissue.

Scrotal Trauma: Recent physical injury involving the scrotum.

Severe Itch: An intense itching sensation that is unbearable.

Severe Pain: Pain that is intolerable, often described as the worst ever. Refer to the chapter on pain assessment for more details.

Shock: A condition marked by insufficient oxygen delivery to tissues, with classic signs including sweating, pallor, tachycardia, hypotension, and reduced consciousness.

Shoulder Tip Pain: Sharp pain located at the tip of the shoulder, often indicating diaphragmatic irritation.

Significant Cardiac History: A history of recurrent life-threatening arrhythmias or any known cardiac condition that may deteriorate rapidly.

Significant Haematological History: A known haematological disorder that has the potential to worsen quickly.

Significant History of Allergy: A documented history of severe allergic reactions, such as to nuts or bee stings.

Significant History of GI Bleed: Any history of major gastrointestinal bleeding or bleeding associated with esophageal varices.

Significant Mechanism of Injury: Injuries from high-energy events like penetrating trauma, high-speed car accidents, or falls from great heights, especially with ejection, fatalities, or vehicle deformation.

Significant Medical History: Pre-existing conditions requiring ongoing medication or specific care.

Significant Psychiatric History: A documented history of a serious psychiatric condition or event.

Significant Respiratory History: A past history of life-threatening respiratory episodes, such as severe COPD or brittle asthma.

Signs of Dehydration: Symptoms include dry tongue, sunken eyes, reduced skin turgor, and in infants, a sunken anterior fontanelle. Usually associated with low urine output.

Signs of Meningism; A stiff neck accompanied by headache and photophobia.

Signs of Moderate Pain: Young children in moderate pain often cry intermittently and are somewhat consolable.

Signs of Severe Pain: Infants or young children in severe pain often

References

1. Altschuld, J. W., & Wang, K. (2020). Triage in the Emergency Department: A Systematic Approach. Journal of Emergency Medicine, 58(4), 467-475.

2. American College of Emergency Physicians (ACEP). (2018). Emergency Severity Index (ESI) Triage Algorithm. ACEP Publishing.

3. Arbabi, S., & Joseph, A. (2017). Critical Care in the Emergency Department: Principles and Practice. Elsevier Health Sciences.

4. Barker, L. M., & Mullan, P. A. (2019). Emergency Triage and Priority Classification. Springer Publishing.

5. Brown, A., & McBride, D. (2016). Trauma Triage: Assessment and Management in the Emergency Department. McGraw-Hill Education.

6. Crandall, M., & LeBlanc, D. (2015). Emergency Nursing: Principles and Practice in Triage and Trauma Care. Wolters Kluwer.

7. Gerdtz, M., & Buckley, T. (2017). Triage: Principles and Practice in Emergency Care. Elsevier Health Sciences.

8. Goff, M. L., & Armstrong, S. (2018). Nursing in Emergency Care: Clinical Skills for the Rapid Assessment and Triage of Patients. Wiley-Blackwell.

9. Hick, J. L., & Barbisch, D. (2018). Disaster Triage: The Role of Emergency Medical Services. Disaster Medicine and Public Health Preparedness, 12(3), 234-241.

10. Hsieh, M., & Saylor, G. (2019). The Emergency Triage Process: Effectiveness and Challenges in Prehospital and Hospital Settings. International Journal of Emergency Medicine, 12(1), 35-41.

11. Jenkins, J. L., & Geyer, T. (2015). Critical Care Nursing: A Holistic Approach to Emergency and Trauma Care. Elsevier.

12. Kerr, J., & Richards, D. (2021). Rapid Assessment and Prioritization in Critical Care: A Comprehensive Guide for Nurses. Oxford University Press.

13. Kissoon, N., & Odetola, F. O. (2020). Triage Systems in Emergency and Trauma Care: The Global Perspective. Springer.

14. Mackway-Jones, K., Marsden, J., & Windle, J. (2016). Advanced Paediatric Life Support: The Practical Approach. BMJ Publishing Group.

15. McLellan, R. (2014). Effective Triage in Emergency Medicine: Making the Right Decisions Under Pressure. McGraw-Hill Education.

16. Nicholson, C., & Connolly, M. (2019). The Role of Triage in Emergency Care: Challenges and Innovations. Journal of Emergency Nursing, 45(2), 112-118.

17. Sills, S., & Martin, L. (2017). Critical Care Nursing: Assessment and Management. Saunders.

18. The National Institute for Health and Care Excellence (NICE). (2020). Emergency and Urgent Care: Principles of Emergency Triage. NICE Guidelines.

19. Triage and Emergency Care Committee of the American Trauma Society. (2017). Triage and Transport Guidelines for Emergency Medical Services. Journal of Trauma Nursing, 24(3), 196-204.

20. Vincent, J. L., & Taccone, F. S. (2019). Critical Care and Emergency Medicine: Current Concepts and Practice. Springer.

21. Walsh, C., & Lee, T. (2018). Advanced Triage Protocols: Improving Outcomes in Emergency and Trauma Care. Cambridge University Press.

22. Wrenn, K., & Johnson, S. (2016). The Role of Triage in Emergency Department Efficiency: Tools and Techniques. Emergency Medicine Clinics of North America, 34(2), 189-202.

23. Wilson, D., & Johnson, R. (2015). Emergency Nursing: Principles and Practice. Pearson Education.

24. Young, D. K., & White, R. L. (2017). Triage Decision Support: Evidence-Based Approaches in Acute Care Settings. Critical Care Nurse, 37(4), 35-43.

www.ingramcontent.com/pod-product-compliance
Lightning Source LLC
Chambersburg PA
CBHW071031240526
45469CB00006BD/2169